Rapid Weight Loss & Deep Sleep Hypnosis (2 in 1): Guided Hypnosis & Meditations For Burning Fat, Food Addiction, Eating Healthy, Insomnia, Falling Asleep Fast, Healing Your Body

By Meditation Made Effortless

Deep Sleep & Rapid Weight Loss Hypnosis: Beginners Guided & Self-Hypnosis For Burning Fat, Overcoming Insomnia, Deep Relaxation Including Positive Affirmations & Meditations

By Meditation Made Effortless

Table of Contents

To the Narrator

The Introduction, Induction, and Deepener should be 30 Min Long

Maintain Sleep Hygiene and Get rid of the thoughts should   be 30 Min long

Eat in Moderation should be 15 Min long

Sugar Addiction be 25 Min long

Letting Go of Labels/Beliefs

should be 25 min long

Further Weight Loss should be 15 min long

Getting Leverage should be 20 min long

Getting Back to Good Health

should be 30 min long

Change Personal History should be 25 min long..

Overcome Insomnia – should be 20 min long

Improving Self Image – should be 20 min long

Insomnia Relaxation should be 15 min long

Affirmations – should be 50 min long

"…" means take a breath while speaking before you continue.

PAUSE (for a few breaths)

LONGER PAUSE (give time to allow the listener time to imagine what you've suggested)

Introduction

Thank you for choosing **Deep Sleep & Rapid Weight Loss Hypnosis audio**...And choosing this audio only means, you have taken a step towards loving yourself even more. Listening to this audio only means you are self-aware of your sleep and weight issues and you want to sleep better and lose weight to be able to feel energetic, positive, and happy. And...hypnosis can get you started on this effortless Deep Sleep and Rapid Weight Loss Journey.

When you are unable to sleep properly or sleep with many awakenings at night, you may feel lethargic, fatigued and irritated the next morning. This also leads to difficulty in concentration and focus.

When you think about the past and worry about the future, which leads to many thoughts when in bed...and it may stop you from falling and staying asleep...

Pause

With changes in the sleep cycle, the body experiences many changes leading to weight gain because lack of sleep leads to changes in hormones that regulate appetite and hunger.

With listening to this audio regularly, you improve the quality of sleep, regularise hormones, and lose weight.

Pause

When you sleep properly, you feel happy and energetic the next day. You are more focused and productive... ultimately leading you to feel motivated and happy. This helps you stay focused and motivated to lose weight and achieve everyday eating and exercise goals to lose weight faster.

So, congratulations on taking this step to overcome sleep and weight issues. Every time you listen to this audio, you get more and more focused on improving the quality of sleep, health, and quality of your life.

I would like you to sit or lay comfortably, where you will not be distracted. Do not listen to this audio when your mind requires your conscious attention.

Pause

Listen to this audio only when you are relaxed and stationary. Please use headphones so that you can focus on the sound of my voice.

Let us start...

Begin recording

Induction

You are now listening to the sound of my voice... and the sound of my voice only ...and as you continue to listen to each word I say...you allow yourself to relax more and more.

Pause

I wonder if you could take a deep breath...hold it for a count of 5... and then exhale.

Pause

Let's start now.

Breathe in Deeply...

Pause

Hold for a count of 5

1... 2...3...4...and 5

Now, exhale...

Pause

Once more, take another deep breath...

Breathe in...

Hold for a count of 5 — 1, 2, 3, 4, 5 (slowly)

Now, breathe out...

Pause

Once more, take another deep breath —

Breathe in

Hold for a count of 5 — 1, 2, 3, 4, 5 (slowly)

Now, breathe out

Pause

And, come back to your normal breathing pattern...

Pause

— And, I wonder... if you could simply bring all your focus and attention to the centre of your eye-brows...with your eyes closed...try to look at the centre of your brows and focus on the point between them...that's right.

Pause

In a moment, I am going to talk to that part of you, which is highly creative...the part that knows exactly how to help you imagine or create anything with the help of your mind's eye.

Pause

And... I know you can do it... because everybody can...we all have a creative mind, that has the ability and capability to create and imagine images in our mind.

I know you must have imagined or visualized or day-dreamed many times in your life. And... our creative part helps us imagine and visualize. Isn't it?

With the help of our creative mind, we can visualize, imagine, write, paint, and dream...and I am going to be talking to that part of you today.

Pause

Deepener

Let your creative part take you on a beautiful journey. The journey that will help you involve all your senses and make you feel you wonderful and much calmer.

Pause

And, I wonder, if you could imagine that you have a private beach, and the whole beach is to yourself. No one else comes to this beach because it belongs to you only.

Longer Pause

You look at the water in front, and notice beautiful waves crashing against the seashore. You listen to the sound of the seagulls….That's right…it's so beautiful and calming.

And, as you look at the waters, you notice many shades of blue, perhaps green too.

You notice light blue, turquoise, deep blue, light green, and several other shades of blue, visible vividly under the beautiful crisp Sunshine….

The sound of the water is soothing to your ears and the sea breeze touches your forehead and cheeks as you walk towards the water on the sand.

Pause

You can feel the water around your ankles and the splashes of water as the waves come crashing against the shore. You move forward and feel the water against your legs…it is soothing and calming.. Isn't it?

You stay inside the water and enjoy the water and Sun…feeling relaxed.

You look towards your right…and notice a comfy hammock tied between two poles. And just on the side, you notice a table with your favourite tropical drink.

Pause

You move towards the hammock to lay in it and relax to enjoy the surroundings as you sip the delicious drink.

Longer Pause

And as you continue to enjoy your drink…you notice a kite in the sky…it's colourful and big perhaps…

You look at it…and it starts to come down towards your beach…

And, as I count down from 10 down to 0, you will find the kite coming closer and closer to the sandy beach and with each count down, you are going to go deeper and deeper into a beautiful state of relaxation.

10...the kite is swaying with the wind

9 ....you are feeling even more relaxed

8...it starts to come closer to the beach

7...you can make out its colours

6 ...as it comes closer...it gets bigger...and you relax yourself even more...

5... you are drifting into a relaxed state of mind

4...deeper and deeper

3...even more relaxed

2...it's going to a touch the beach in a moment

1...its fallen on the beach

0...you are beautifully and deeply relaxed.

Maintain Sleep Hygiene Script

Sleep comes to people naturally and it is a normal process for everyone... You used to sleep peacefully when you were a baby. You learnt a process where you could not sleep properly or perhaps woke up many times during the night...

Pause

The time has come to change this pattern and go back to the old self who used to sleep like a baby and enjoy the sleep. And, for this, you may have to learn habits that are important for you to sleep better without any disturbance at night.

Pause

You know the importance of sleep and how deep sleep and good quality sleep can improve the quality of your life. Isn't it?

With better sleep, you are relaxed, energised, positive, and happy that ultimately improves the quality of the relationship with yourself and the quality of your life.

Pause

From today on...you limit your day time naps to 30 minutes and this helps you sleep better at night. If you wish to sleep during the day to feel fresh...you put an alarm in the day for 30 minutes only. You do not resist the sleep, but be disciplined around it and put a 30 minute alarm to feel alert and fresh.

And I wonder if you know the importance of physical exercising in promoting sleep...

You exercise regularly for at least 30 minutes to feel happy, lose weight and to promote sleep. You avoid strenuous workouts post 8 pm.

You avoid stimulants like alcohol and caffeine after 6 pm. Because they make the brain active and stop you from falling asleep...

You avoid eating heavy meals just before going to bed. You finish your food by 8 pm and if at all you feel hungry post that you have a warm glass of milk. Milk promotes sleep whether animal or almond milk.

You maintain a regular bedtime and keep your phone away. You make a habit of writing all your worries in a worry journal...for not more than 10 minutes and when you close that you know you are ready to let go and sleep.

Pause

You take enough Sunlight to regularise the sleep wake cycle.

You make sure that your sleep environment is calming and pleasant...you ensure that the lights are dim with black out curtains.

Longer Pause.

And as you maintain this sleep hygiene everyday...it gets easier and easier for you to fall asleep every night and staying asleep.

You prepare yourself every night...one hour before going to bed...perhaps you drink warm milk, take a warm shower, massage your feet with warm oil, write your worries in worry journal...and keep your phone far away...

With every passing day...you are getting in the habit of maintaining sleep hygiene to improve the quantity and quality of your sleep..

Longer Pause

Get Rid of the Thoughts and Sleep Better

And, I wonder if you can imagine that there is a room somewhere in your mind, a brightly lit room. Perhaps there's a window through... which the sunshine is coming. And... you notice the room to be full of thoughts and with so much light, you can easily see the thoughts on the walls and the ceiling. They are all there on the four walls...when you look at each side.

You notice them as graffiti or posters or banners...

Longer Pause

Perhaps these are the thoughts from the past about the events that have already happened a long time ago...or perhaps from the latest time.

Pause

On the floor you notice thoughts about the future...and these are mere worries that are not really under your control. But somehow you know that these thoughts about the past and future keep you up and stop you from falling asleep on time.

And, you know with so much on the walls and ceiling, you are getting distracted. You cannot peacefully sit and sleep in the room, because it is full of so many things that are keeping you distracted from the present day.

The time has come to change everything in the room so that you are not distracted and you can sit or sleep peacefully...

Because you want to sleep...isn't it?

I know you can do that...because everybody can.

In a moment, you will notice that there is a staircase for you to reach the top of the walls and ceiling easily. And, just on the side of the staircase, you notice a big trash can to put the posters and banners...and on the other side of the staircase...you notice big buckets of black paint...with a big paint brush.

And, with your powerful imagination...you get on the staircase and reach the ceiling and walls to take off the posters and banners of thoughts from past and future...they do not serve any purpose...they only keep you up for long or give you many awakenings at night, making you feel fatigued the next day and also...making you gain weight.

With all this, you have decided to take them off and put them in the trash can. Isn't it?

Start the job, take off the banners, posters, and put them in the trash can.

Longer Pause

And as you do that...you feel some weight has been lifted off your body and you instantly feel relaxed and calm.

Pause

There are no banners and posters on the walls, but some text or graffiti on the walls. These can be taken off by painting the walls black.

Pick up the brush and start painting the walls black...and as you do that...you feel the sense of relaxation and calm taking over all your senses...

You start to feel relaxed and calm...with every paint stroke....

Colour the walls black now.

Longer Pause

The room is now painted black, the window is shut, and there is no light coming in.

You now look at the floor and you notice future worries ....these are the words that make you anxious or worrisome...and these also keep you up at night...or stop you from falling asleep.

You now need to scrub the floor to get rid of all that you see...

There is a bucket of water and soap....with a scrubber...

You now get to the work...and scrub off all that you see on the floor....

With every stroke…you are getting rid of two worries…that's right…

You can clean the floor now….

Longer Pause

The room now looks absolutely clean from all sides…

It's comfy and you are not distracted…

You now allow yourself to count back from 5 down to 0…and with each count down…you will be twice as relaxed and twice as deep.

5…feeling relaxed
4…going deeper and deeper
3…relaxing more and more..
2…entering a deep state of relaxation
1…calmer and deeper

Affirmations for Sleep

I would now like you to repeat the suggestions after me..

It's easier for me to let go every night (4-5 seconds pause)

I close my eyes and paint the room black when I want to sleep (4-5 seconds pause)

With every brush stroke, it's easier for me to let go and drift into a peaceful sleep (4-5 seconds pause)

I feel drowsier when you imagine yourself painting the room black (4-5 seconds pause)

My mind is relaxed and my thoughts slow down as soon as I hit the bed (4-5 seconds pause)

Eat in Moderation

And, I wonder if you can look at your eating habits...and I wonder if you can simply relax and enjoy the lightness of your body and mind...

I wonder if you know that our stomachs are built to take in food that can fit into our palms but we eat more and let it expand so much that it craves for bigger meals, making us eat more calories and making us gain weight.

Pause

We all are born with a natural ability to know when we are full and our bodies give us signals when we know we are full.

But we ignore these signals because we get caught up in talking, eating, watching movies while eating.

Pause

And because we are not mindful of our eating and get busy doing something else along with that.... we pay attention to other things and rarely give attention to our body's signal.

This makes us eat more and we overeat...expanding our stomachs...making us gain weight...looking thicker and chubbier...

And, now is the time to change this... to be able to reach your ideal goal weight, feel lighter, look slimmer, fitter, and confident. Isn't it?

I wonder if you can imagine the recent time when you overate and how you felt..

Go back to that time now...

Pause

And as you are there...imagine and visualise how you are feeling as you overeat...can you feel the palpitations...and the stuffy feelings...and then how do you feel after eating extra?

Perhaps guilty…

And imagine if you continue to overstuff yourself in every meal and continue to feel guilty…how would you see yourself three months from now?

Longer Pause

Get to know your emotional and physical health…is it getting better or deteriorating?

But you won't reach this state…because you are listening to me and this only means that you want to stop this old habit of yours and eat in moderation.

You can program your mind to eat a healthy and right amount of food where you feel full and not eat extra.

And your very powerful subconscious mind knows exactly when to signal you when you have eaten enough. I wonder if you can now go within yourself and ask your mind to alert you when you have eaten enough that is enough for the body for it to survive and thrive.

Longer Pause

And, as you continue to listen to me…with every word I say…and with every word you hear… you allow yourself to note everything that your subconscious mind is telling you.

All the messages that it is giving and the signals that you will know that you have eaten enough…you know now. And you will listen to this signal…and the message given to you by your subconscious mind. You are now being aware of the signal consciously and subconsciously and this reminds you to stop eating.

Longer Pause

The more you listen to it, the better control you have on this habit and it gets effortless and easier for you to lose weight.

Affirmations/Suggestions

Repeat the below suggestions in your mind after me…

I am aware of the signal to stop eating when I have eaten enough (4-5 seconds pause)

I stop eating when I get the signal (4-5 seconds pause)

I eat mindfully (4-5 seconds pause)

I chew my food at least 10 times in my mouth (4-5 seconds pause)

I relish all the tastes and flavours of each mouthful (4-5 seconds pause)

I love myself and with every passing day I am getting slimmer and slimmer (4-5 seconds pause)

Sugar Addiction

You are listening to me because you are aware of the positive effects of weight loss and you want to achieve the target weight goal. Isn't it?

And one of the ways to promote weight loss and lose weight faster is to give up on sugar. Sugar may make you happy when you have it because it releases dopamine and you want to continue to feel good so you reach the jar of cookies or cakes sitting in the refrigerator more often than required.

Pause

While it makes you happy it has long term effects on your health and you do not want to suffer permanently because something gives you pleasure temporarily. Isn't it?

If you continue to have sugar, it will not only make you gain weight but will affect your mood and brain function. In addition, it will affect your teeth and other organs like kidney, liver, pancreas, and skin.

According to research, the more sugar you eat, the more you will weigh and people who drink sugary beverages tend to weigh more and are at a higher risk of type 2 diabetes. This is because excess amounts of sugar can expand fat cells that releases chemicals leading to weight gain.

And you want to be free and lead a healthy life where you see yourself as slim, fit, and light...isn't it?

And, I wonder if you can imagine or visualise that you are continuing to eat sugar and have sugary drinks for three more months....and I wonder if you can imagine yourself three months from now?

Longer Pause

Have you gained more weight? Look at your legs, stomach, and shoulders...are they looking bulkier. And, now look at yourself six months from now if you continue to have sugary foods and drinks.

Even more bulkier? Look at your teeth and perhaps your skin...

Longer Pause

The good news is that you do not have to face all this because this is when you continue to have sugar but you are listening to me to let go of sugar addiction and this means you will never reach this time in future...and perhaps you will look completely opposite after six months.

Now is the time for you to take control and responsibility for what you do and don't put into your body. You only have this one body and if you damage it for good...you will not be able to pop to the shops and get a new one.

And, now you will change the way you look and think about sugar. And, I want you to fully focus on this experience so that you are able to change the experience and relationship with the sugar.

Pause

Continue to focus on the sound of my voice and the sound of my voice only. And, in the future, you will find sugar disgusting and you no longer want to eat it. The only way to stop having sugar is to completely cut the sugar intake or drinks with added sugar completely.

And listening to this only makes you feel empowered and you know you can reach your ideal goal weight faster if you completely get rid of sugary foods and drinks.

And, I wonder if you can think of your favourite sugary food that you love. And, imagine putting that in your mouth and as you chew it...you know it's getting melted in your mouth and sticking to your teeth and tongue...and you can feel the layer of scum on your teeth, which starts to decay them...and your teeth feel unhappy and sick.

Pause

You feel like getting rid of it...but it is difficult to do so...it just can't come off...and then some of it gets stuck in your saliva...and perhaps... because of stickiness...you also feel a strand of hair and I don't know whose hair is it...but you can feel it ...mixed up with that...and it's in your throat...and you can't get rid of it...and it is making you choke and gag...and you are truly disgusted.

And, you choke and gag...and in a moment...and you can taste sugar, someone's hair...and the choking feeling...

And, I am going to count down from 5 down 0...with each count down...the choking feeling, taste, and the thought of hair...would fade...with each count down.

5, 4, 3, 2, 1, 0....

5...the feeling and taste are diminishing
4...it's fading
3...you are feeling comfortable
2...you are relaxed..
1...you are giving up sugar...
0...you have given up sugar..

And now, every time you see your favourite sugary stuff, you know that eating that will give you the same feelings of choking, gaging, the thought of someone's hair will come in your mind...and you will stop and distract your mind to something else. Perhaps to natural sugars...found in fruits.

Letting Go of Labels/Beliefs

And as you continue to listen to each word I say and continue to go deeper and deeper into a beautiful state of relaxation... I would like you to look within you and look for that place where you have all labels stored. Labels about yourself.

Perhaps the labels that you created or the labels you believed in because others believed in them about you...and those labels that were given to you by others.

Look for those labels...perhaps they are positive and negative.. Perhaps they are compliments or comments...look within yourself and find them now.

Longer Pause

And as you continue to go deeper and deeper, it gets easier to locate them...and I want you to find all the beliefs related to weight loss or weight gain or body...

I know you can do it because everybody can...

And I remember having a conversation with someone I knew who was a therapist and she had a conversation with her father who had a belief that it's difficult to lose weight...and even though he tried all the diets, changed relationship with food, exercised, he could not lose much weight... because the belief or the label he had given to himself was its difficult to lose weight and I cannot lose weight.

And with talking to my friend, he became aware of the limiting belief or label and got rid of it...and then the place it was residing, he filled it up with a positive label or belief that I can lose weight easily... safely...and effortlessly.

Longer Pause

And the real problem was having this belief and I wonder if you have something similar and if yes, then the time has come to get rid of it..

Just imagine getting rid of it ...perhaps in the form of a banner or label coming out of your body and reaching a cloud up above... imagine the cloud absorbing it...going millions of millions of miles away...

As it goes up...you feel lighter and lighter...and you know that it's going to be so easy to lose weight with regular exercise and eating right.

And...you fill up the place with a positive label that it's going to be so much easier for you to lose weight now..

Perhaps it's : I lose weight easily or I can lose weight..

Whatever label or belief you want to put yourself in...do that now...

Longer Pause.

And, repeat it five times in your mind....

Longer Pause

That's right...you are now focused and motivated to achieve your ideal goal weight..

Your thoughts, emotions, and actions are working together and harmoniously for you to achieve what you want to achieve...the ideal goal weight...

And, I wonder if you could imagine...yourself three months from now...having achieved a fitter and slimmer body..

What do you notice?

Look at your face, your chest, and your legs...

See how slim you have gotten...and feeling so much lighter and happier...isn't it?

And you can do this and achieve this body knowing and believing that you can lose weight, easily.

You don't try to lose weight...you lose weight.

Affirmations/Suggestions

And, I wonder if you can repeat the following in your mind to strengthen the belief that you are losing weight..

- I am losing weight

- I lose weight easily

- Weight loss is easy

- I can do it

- Every day I am even more motivated to achieve weight loss goals

- I am getting fitter and slimmer

Further Weight loss

You continue to listen to the sound of my voice and the sound of my voice only. And from now on, you will use food only when you are physically hungry and not when you are emotionally or mentally hungry.

You know that food cannot be used in place of an emotion and when you are sad... to feel happy, you substitute happiness with food...and you know that it will only give you negative emotions later, which is guilt or regret.

Do you want to get into that vicious cycle?

Pause

To stay out of the vicious cycle, you always need to make a conscious decision when you are choosing to eat food. Always become aware of the thought and see what it says before you take any action.

You eat to live and to give nutrients to your body and not to give love to your heart or mind.

You eat smaller meals throughout the day...perhaps six smaller meals and exercise regularly to increase the metabolism.

When you are hungry at odd times, you fill yourself up with water based drinks like water or lemonade or black coffee.

You love healthy and nutritious food and look forward to eating meals with plenty of vegetables and fruits. And you plan your meals beforehand so that you know what you are going to eat for each meal. This gives you plenty of energy to move through the day.

Longer Pause

Eating right and exercising also promotes sleep... which in turn promotes weight loss.

And as you continue to achieve goals and you start to notice significant changes in your body shape and weight...with every passing week...

You start to look fitter and better and your clothes fit you even better.

Perhaps with this, you may even think of changing your wardrobe completely with smaller sizes and clothes that are aligned with the latest fashion.

And, I want you to imagine doing that now...Imagine changing your wardrobe with smaller sizes and fashionable clothes.

Longer Pause

With this, you are even more prepared to stay focused on your weight loss journey. You easily say no to sugary and fried foods and say yes to healthy foods with natural sugars.

The more nutritious and healthier foods you eat, the better you feel with every passing day and get excited to plan the meals for the next day.

Pause

And as you continue to plan and eat healthy meals, you can see you are becoming slimmer and more attractive...and perhaps getting ready for a beach holiday.

As soon as you look at the variety of foods, you know what to choose and what to leave. You are easily able to eliminate the foods that make you fat, lousy, lazy, and affect your body weight and skin.

Pause

You choose and pick those foods that make you remember your best body that you want to achieve. The moment you look at healthy foods, you will get an image of you in your mind at your ideal goal weight, wearing attractive clothes.

And it would be easier for you to overlook the unhealthy foods.

Pause

With every passing day, you notice your hair getting better, skin getting better, stomach and thighs getting slimmer and smaller.

And you know you can achieve all this by rejecting all the unhealthy foods and focus on healthy and nutritious foods.

Weight Loss- Getting Leverage.

Now, it is very clear to you...that it takes a certain amount of motivation to make this work. But in order to get the best out of your investment of time and money, there needs to be a lot more of this desire to work towards your goal...

It comes upon you to choose to stop treating your body like an indispensable dumping ground. You see the signs your body is giving you... that it won't put up with this forever. A warning of your unhealthy lifestyles is your tummy. How much longer will it take for you to see these signs?

Over the course of time, we have all suffered the loss of someone. Even though they are gone, we realize that they were an important part of our life... You need to take a look at people who love and care for you...people who hold you dear and rely on you to be there when they need you.

Longer Pause

It is your sole purpose to ensure that they do not suffer the loss of a loved one. It becomes you responsibility to live a healthy, long life with love and respect for your body.... Appreciate the gift of life by choosing to eat healthy, in the right amount and at the right time rather than food that harms you.

Longer Pause

Here I understand that nobody likes being told what to do; so I won't tell you of the dangers you bring upon your life by being overweight...

I won't tell you that overeating greasy food is dangerous and prevents you from having your desired slim, beautiful healthy body.

I will not note down that every fried and sweet food has a high fat and calorie rate that takes away the pleasure of eating it. I would rather just ask you to see yourself if you make the healthy choices and understand how it will make you feel as you make these choices now.

Longer Pause

Body Getting back to Good Health

What do you see when you look yourself in the mirror? Do you see yourself as you are, the real you or it is an image prompted by a chain of thought you built up as a product of your mind conditioning and experiences...

Irrespective of the answer that comes to you now after a deep thought, I am here to let you know that the way you see yourself is going to change for the better...

Pause

It will cleanse and refresh you like a gentle cool breeze only to improve the quality of life. The cobwebs that mask your beauty and your abilities will be blown away.

Your confidence to be able to develop, grow and become stronger by the minute will be brought back into the light.

Let us begin with you focusing on your body. Try to see and understand that your body is nature's miracle. Try to spot a plant or tree that can heal or cause a change in its body by thinking positively.

But the life that you have has given you the ability to cause an effect on your body parts simply by thinking about it, to make it better or worse. You have the ability to earn whatever you set your mind on with a bit of focus.

Notice that when you think of buying a new car, you not only visualize the way it looks but also see how it is being driven around. Your body also has a similar way.

Longer Pause

When something goes wrong, it suddenly doesn't become enough to discard it and think "I don't want this illness anymore . . . " or "I want to stop worrying about my ailments". This only leads to your mind picking up in the positives of these statements, turning and twisting them into "I want this illness." and "I want to worry."

From this moment onwards, start reviewing and censoring any thoughts that come to your mind or any words that come out of your mouth.

Comprehend only the positives and focus on what you wish to achieve. Make sure that every day, you are telling yourself that "My body is returning to natural health" and "My body takes care of me.

You don't realise the numerous functions and skills your body controls unconsciously. These simple functions such as blinking, walking and talking come naturally to you. But the more you think about it the more unfamiliar they begin to feel.

As you focus on these oddities and unfamiliarity, it creates a sense of uneasiness that very soon escalates to paranoia and later causes stress responses from all body parts.

Longer Pause

Grasp the fact that your body takes it upon itself to rejuvenate automatically, and it does this best when you rest and relax.

The more relaxed you feel, the more rest you get, the better it works on its natural functions.

So in the coming week, forget of any problems that you might have and be amazed by the way you feel when you are properly relaxed.

Change Personal History

As you allow yourself to go deeper and deeper, I would like you to know that…

You have the ability to take charge of your life and have full control over it. You are capable and have the ability to be your ideal goal weight in the desired time.

In order to ensure that there is no further relapse, take a look back at your very first attempt and locate the first incident, a comment or any other trigger that caused you to loose belief and confidence in your weight loss journey.

Longer Pause

It might seem to be something insignificant, so as to go unnoticed by you back then. Now, you need to take a closer look and find the root of the problem that changed your entire perspective on any further attempts of your journey to the body you desire.

Once you find and eliminate this issue, nothing stands between you and your determination to succeed.

First, try and locate your most recent experience where you lacked the confidence in your ability to losing weight.

I know you can find it…because everybody can…

Pause

Recollect where you were at this moment, what you were doing and who you were with. Pay attention to anything said or done by you or anyone around you that might have caused this reaction in you.

I want you to put yourself back in that situation and this time offer yourself some kind, encouraging words. Talk to your past self and make them believe in their self. Give them the confidence and the encouragement they lack in order to succeed.

Give them reasons to keep going, not to give up or sabotage any of their efforts. Offer them some comfort, wise words or perhaps a different perspective to change his/her feelings and behaviour.

Pause

Now grab your past self by the shoulders and tell him/her "You can do this.", as you look him/her in the eyes. As you say this, feel it and believe it through every fibre in your body.

And when you are satisfied that you have truly enforced the belief to never give up, move back further into the bridge of time to the next similar event where you lost hope and gave up.

Stand with your past self again; repeat the paragraph to ensure hope and confidence in this event. We will now take a few minutes as you continue to travel to all such points of significant incidences, repairing and reassuring yourself as you make the necessary changes. You need to offer advice and comfort to correct every situation that might have sabotaged your efforts.

Longer Pause

Now visualize a situation in the future where you might stray from your goals. Step into that picture in front of yourself and tell him/her to stop. Coach yourself the way you have in the past. Reason with yourself to stay focused and committed to your goal.

Longer Pause

Do it for this supposed situation and then do it again if you can think of any more situations where you might run off track.

Repeat the reasons to stay strong, believing in your words of encouragement and do not give up unless you have convinced yourself not to drift away from your path to success.

With this, you have moulded a powerful tool in and as yourself. It is okay to make a few mistakes in your journey. A real achievement comes with its ups and downs. Even an arrow shot to hit the bull's eye trebles in its path as it cuts through air.

Pause

It is fine if you under achieve because as you look back on the long way you've come, you see that you have done well and have come very far and this gives you the courage to keep flying unless you hit the bull's eye.

Overcome Insomnia

And as you continue to listen to each word I say, I wonder if you can imagine a beautiful white fluffy cloud just beneath you…and you notice yourself laying comfortably on it.

In a moment, you notice that it starts to gently drift and you are drifting along with it…

Feeling lighter, calmer, and relaxed…

And this cloud is the depiction of relaxation, comfort, and calmness…

Pause

Every time, you want to sleep…simply imagine drifting away with the cloud….away from the physical world…into a world of relaxation and calmness…

That's right.

And as you continue to listen to me, you allow yourself to drift further and further away…finding yourself to be sleepier and drowsier…

And the more you feel drowsier…the more your body feels relaxed and you go twice as deep into a beautiful state of relaxation…

Pause

You are now comfortably relaxed and your physical body is at rest…

And as you continue to enjoy the beautiful state of relaxation, you notice that this cloud has a special power to absorb every little worry that you may have…that bothers you and stops you from falling asleep..

Pause

The cloud begins to absorb every little worry and as that happens…you notice the cloud becoming heavier and heavier….turns darker and darker…and you begin to feel lighter and lighter…

That's right.

Send all your tensions and worries about your past and future to this large cloud…

It can take all of it in…

Leaving you feeling light and free…

Pause

With every little tension and worry it absorbs, get closer and closer to the sleep….and you can feel the bedding beneath your body…

The comfortable mattress and the bed sheet…and the very comfy pillow…

It is so cosy and relaxing and every time you rest your head on the pillow…you imagine the cloud above your head….and it starts to drift…away into the deepest state of relaxation..

And, you start to give it the day's worries and tension to the cloud…and the cloud takes all of that in…making you feel calmer and free…to help you fall asleep…

Pause

If there are any residual worries…you may imagine the same room with the graffiti, texts, and banner…and you start to paint the walls in black…

And with every stroke of black paint brush…your erase the graffiti…texts…banners…and the thoughts get painted with black…

The room gets darker and darker…and you feel calmer and calmer…

All the residual thoughts from past and future…

Paint them all..

Longer Pause

And in a moment…I am going to count you down from 10 down to 0…and with each count down…your will be painting the room black…and entering a deep state of relaxation…

10….strokes of paint on the walls…

9…the paint covers the thoughts well…

8…you cannot make out what is behind the paint

7…the room is getting darker..

6…you are thoughtless…

5…you allow yourself to drift further into the state of slumber

4…going further deep

3…drifting even more…

2...becoming even more relaxed

1 ...about to sleep

0...deep sleep...

Improve Self-Image

And as you continue to listen to me and allow yourself to drift more and more into a beautiful state of relaxation, I wonder if your mind is open to my suggestions that will have a positive effect on your mind and body.

Pause

You are a great human being with many qualities that your real self is happy, lively, fun, contented...but lately...it all got fogged with eating more...which is inflicting emotional pain.

You know that with eating more you feel guilty and think why did you eat more or eat unhealthy...so you again take actions to eat to feel better...and then feel guilty...this is a never ending vicious cycle...causing you emotional pain.

And...because of this... there is a fog of guilt and other negative thoughts that have stopped you from seeing who you truly are. Isn't it?

I know you are very intelligent and you have the capability to be self-aware...and that is why you are listening to me because you are self-aware of your weight and the goal you want to achieve. That certainly makes you wise and intelligent.

Pause

And, I know you would know that self-love and better appearance come from the states of mind rather than using superficial products to look better. If you believe in yourself and choose not to focus on negative thoughts, you will always want to do better for yourself.

A person who thinks they are ugly or not good enough would always sabotage their efforts to improvise themselves.

If you feel good enough and feel happy, you are in a better frame of mind to achieve weight loss goals and feel the two states of mind – to feel good and look good are always working together harmoniously in your mind.

Pause

So, the better you feel, the better you look and the better you look, the better you feel. Your outside is the reflection of your inside...and better you feel from inside, it is going to reflect on your outside...

And when you see it on your outside and when others see it on your outside...you feel great...you feel appreciated by yourself and others...and then you feel even better...

The more confident you feel, the happier you feel...it's is going to reflect on your body...and you will be even more motivated to achieve your ideal goal weight.

With every passing day, you use your intelligence and be aware of your thoughts...and you choose to focus on the thoughts that make you feel better...and the thoughts that serve no purpose...you simply say "Delete" to those thoughts in your mind...or perhaps show the stop sign to those thoughts...and shift your focus to the positive thoughts...

Longer Pause

And with this, you continue to feel good and continue to look good...and all this reflects on your skin, body, and you stay focused on your weight loss journey.

Insomnia Relaxation

Relaxing your body becomes the first step when you wish to sleep. Let each part of your body relax bit by bit, moving upwards from your toe to your feet, the ankles, the legs, the waist, the chest, the shoulders, your back, arms, hands, throat and then finally your facial muscles....

Pause

As your body relaxes completely, place yourself on a beautiful staircase taking you down to your special place, making you more relaxed, calmer and sleepier.

Keep on counting as you spiral down the stairs and watch everything else dwindle as you reach down to the bottom. Allow your mind to relax in this special, private place. This special place can be envisioned to be anything - from a tropical beach to a simple beautiful sunset. Imagine a warm, comfortable mist surrounding you and let your mind wander wherever it will go.

Longer Pause

Observe your mind as a distant observer as it pulls out images from your subconscious. Watch these images as they gently and softly drift up floating before you.

Feel yourself floating to a comfortable place with your mind and let yourself feel safe, secure and happy in this relaxing feeling. Sink deeper into wherever your mind takes you as you start feeling sleepier and more relaxed than ever before.

Pause

You are now going to start drifting into a short sleep. For now, imagine a soft mist going into your special place and watch it as it grows thicker, warmer becoming more pleasant and comfortable by the minute.

Pause

As you listen to the sound of my voice allowing this mist to surround you, notice all your thoughts, feelings and memories drifting in and out of your awareness. As the most envelopes your entire self, all of your thoughts, feelings and memories become vague and my voice become more distant, dimming and fading away.

You notice how some vague thoughts and ideas try and enter your consciousness until they finally clear out of your mind with time. Let all these thoughts come up and sit tight as these fade away slowly with my voice.

Hear my sound becoming lower and then disappearing all at once. You now find yourself gliding into a light, comfortable space deep within yourself. You are now going to sleep for a short while as my voice becomes less and less clear. After some time, you are going to hear my voice calling out your name to help you come out of this sleep and return to a comfortable hypnotic rest for a brief time.

Pause

You are now drifting into a deep, diffusing, hazy state of rest; slowly and comfortably falling asleep.

Pause

You have done well. From now onwards, you can drift away into sleep when you wish to. Float into the state of hypnotic rest reaching into your special place. Drain out anything that tenses your body as your body is shrouded by a warm, heavy and comfortable mist.

Any thoughts and memories gliding into your consciousness slowly fade away while you drift into sleep. Sleep for as long as you need to and return back to repeat this process if disturbed at any moment.

Affirmations/Suggestions

1. You nourish your body with healthy food (7 seconds pause)

2. You are full of vitality and energy (7 seconds pause)

3. You love to exercise because it makes you happy (7 seconds pause)

4. You are releasing weight effortlessly (7 seconds pause)

5. You are willing to change (7 seconds pause)

6. You let go of the past easily (7 seconds pause)

7. You are getting energetic with every passing day (7 seconds pause)

8. You pay attention to your sleep (7 seconds pause)

9. I am strong and healthy. (7 seconds pause)

10. You drink at least eight glasses of water everyday (7 seconds pause)

11. You look forward to your daily workout sessions. (7 seconds pause)

12. You listen to the signal and stop when you have eaten enough (7 seconds pause)

13. You are healthy and happy (7 seconds pause)

14. You love to exercise everyday (7 seconds pause)

15. You love to eat fruits and vegetables everyday (7 seconds pause)

16. You are becoming stronger and slimmer with every passing day (7 seconds pause)

17. When you crave sugar, you eat natural foods (7 seconds pause)

18. You are grateful for your health (7 seconds pause)

19. You are practice gratitude everyday (7 seconds pause)

20. You are open to new ways of eating (7 seconds pause)

21. You choose food that make your body stronger and healthier (7 seconds pause)

22. You chew food slowly (7 seconds pause)

23. You relish each mouthful and chew food at least 10 times (7 seconds pause)

24. You are becoming slimmer and lighter every day (7 seconds pause)

25. You love your body and mind (7 seconds pause)

26. You enjoy taking care of your body and mind (7 seconds pause)

27. You maintain sleep hygiene everyday (7 seconds pause)

28. You limit your day time naps to 30 minutes (7 seconds pause)

29. You can do it (7 seconds pause)

30. You are flexible (7 seconds pause)

31. You listen to your body (7 seconds pause)

32. You eat in moderation (7 seconds pause)

33. You eat wholesome foods (7 seconds pause)

34. You leave your past behind (7 seconds pause)

35. You feel decisive and enthusiastic (7 seconds pause)

36. You love your life (7 seconds pause)

37. You set everyday sleep and weight loss goals (7 seconds pause)

38. You take everyday actions to achieve goals (7 seconds pause)

39. You are motivated (7 seconds pause)

40. You focus on the good (7 seconds pause)

41. You are grateful (7 seconds pause)

42. You are happy (7 seconds pause)

43. You are self-aware (7 seconds pause)

44. You love the taste of healthy food (7 seconds pause)

45. You are grateful for the foods that make you healthy (7 seconds pause)

46. All the weights and burdens from the past are melting away (7 seconds pause)

47. You are getting leaner and lighter (7 seconds pause)

48. You are getting fitter and slimmer (7 seconds pause)

49. You see beauty in your body (7 seconds pause)

50. You learn new ways easily (7 seconds pause)

51. Your body is getting healed (7 seconds pause)

52. Everyday you wake up you have feelings of gratitude (7 seconds pause)

53. You trust the process of life (7 seconds pause)

54. You trust yourself and trust your body (7 seconds pause)

55. You love yourself (7 seconds pause)

56. You are compassionate towards yourself (7 seconds pause)

57. You eat mindfully and enjoy every mouthful (7 seconds pause)

58. You are balanced (7 seconds pause)

59. You are competent and capable. (7 seconds pause)

60. You are worthy of love and care (7 seconds pause)

61. You give all the love and care to your own body first (7 seconds pause)

62. You choose positive thoughts (7 seconds pause)

63. You are blessed and abundant (7 seconds pause)

64. You love yourself unconditionally (7 seconds pause)

65. You are complete and whole. (7 seconds pause)

66. You are confident and courageous (7 seconds pause)

67. You forgive yourself for all the past mistakes (7 seconds pause)

68. You stay in present and are more mindful (7 seconds pause)

69. You are confident (7 seconds pause)

70. You have high self esteem (7 seconds pause)

71. You are losing weight every day (7 seconds pause)

72. You are focused on your weight loss journey (7 seconds pause)

73. You pay attention to your food intake (7 seconds pause)

74. You chew your food many times (7 seconds pause)

75. You maintain sleep hygiene (7 seconds pause)

76. You love yourself unconditionally (7 seconds pause)

77. Your body is getting fitter and slimmer (7 seconds pause)

78. You are successful (7 seconds pause)

79. You are confident and motivated (7 seconds pause)

80. You believe in yourself (7 seconds pause)

81. You are good enough (7 seconds pause)

82. You enjoy healthy foods (7 seconds pause)

83. You do pleasurable activities everyday (7 seconds pause)

84. You are intelligent and wise (7 seconds pause)

85. You are lovable, open to receive and give love (7 seconds pause)

86. You enjoy your life (7 seconds pause)

87. You enjoy healthy food (7 seconds pause)

88. You have a beautiful relationship with food and your body (7 seconds pause)

Rapid Weight Loss Hypnosis For Women: Beginners Guided Meditations & Self-Hypnosis For Burning Fat, Overcoming Food Addiction, Eating Healthy Including Positive Affirmations

By Meditation Made Effortless

Table of Contents

"..." means take a breath while speaking before you continue.

PAUSE (for a few breaths)

LONGER PAUSE (give time to allow the listener time to imagine what you've suggested)

Introduction

Thank you for picking up the Rapid Weight Loss for women hypnosis audio... this surely is a sign of self-love and it only means that you want to burn fat and slim down...to be able to feel and look great. And...hypnosis can get you started on this effortless weight loss journey.

Pause

So, congratulations for taking this step towards a fitter and happier YOU...please listen to this audio using headphones... so that the sound of my voice is clear and if you lose track of me and your mind starts to wander...you can easily tune back into the sound of my voice.

Pause

Do not listen to this audio...when your mind needs you to be conscious such as while operating machinery or driving. Listen to this audio... when you are in a comfortable position...sitting on a chair or resting on a bed.

Pause

One last note, hypnotherapists usually work with their patients for 6-12 sessions to achieve lasting results with Weight Loss hypnotherapy, therefore, we recommend you go through these Hypnosis around 6-12 times over the next couple of weeks/ months, ideally commit to several chapters of this book each day.

However, each situation is unique and can depend on you, your mental state and the intensity of change you want to being into your life. Therefore, while we offer 6-12 sessions as a recommendation, this is not set in stone and you may need more or less. After each set of sessions, see how you feel, and then decide if you need more.

We also recommend sticking to one set of recordings over a period of time, rater than chopping and changing. For example, you may also have our Sleep Hypnosis, but we recommend completing this one, fully first before moving on to that one.

Now, sit back and relax, it's time to get started.

Let us start... 5 Minutes

Begin recording

Induction

You are now listening to the sound of my voice... and the sound of my voice only ...and as you continue to listen to each word I say...you allow yourself to relax more and more.

Pause

I wonder if you could take a deep breath...hold it for a count of 5... and then exhale.

Pause

Let's start now.

Breathe in Deeply...

Pause

Hold for a count of 5

1... 2...3...4...and 5

Now, exhale...
Pause

Once more, take another deep breath...

Breathe in...

Hold for a count of 5 — 1, 2, 3, 4, 5 (slowly)

Now, breathe out...
Pause

Once more, take another deep breath —

Breathe in

Hold for a count of 5 — 1, 2, 3, 4, 5 (slowly)

Now, breathe out

Pause

And, come back to your normal breathing pattern...

Pause

— And, I wonder… if you could simply bring all your focus and attention to the center of your eye-brows…with your eyes closed…try to look at the center of your brows and focus on the point between them…that's right.

Pause

In a moment, I am going to talk to that part of you, which is highly creative…the part that knows exactly how to help you imagine or create anything with the help of your mind's eye.

Pause

And… I know you can do it… because everybody can…we all have a creative mind, that has the ability and capability to create and imagine images in our mind.

I know you must have imagined or visualized or day-dreamed many times in your life. And… our creative part helps us imagine and visualize. Isn't it?

With the help of our creative mind, we can visualize, imagine, write, paint, and dream…and I am going to be talking to that part of you today.

Pause

Deepener

And, I wonder if that part of you can help you imagine... that you are laying on a beautiful grass, the grass is moist, and you can feel the wonderful moist grass beneath your feet...

Longer Pause (8 seconds pause)

The day is beautiful, the Sun is shining bright... and you can feel the warm sunshine touch your skin gently...

Pause

As you look around, you notice there are bushes and trees around you... and perhaps a stream of water somewhere nearby as you hear the magical sound of the water flowing...

Pause

There's a beautiful fragrance of flowers around you...and you can smell the fragrance of your favorite flowers... as you continue to imagine that, I wonder if you can notice a tree next to you. A tall tree...with many branches and green leaves having different shades of green...And, as you notice the trunk of the tree, you notice a black ant moving down the trunk to reach its roots visible just above the ground.

The tree seems quite old and strong...

You focus on it... and with every little distance it covers down the trunk...you find yourself drifting more and more and falling deeper and deeper into a beautiful state of relaxation...

Pause

Starting now...

10... Look at the movement of the ant

9 ...see how it moves down the tree trunk

8 ... drifting down and down

7 ... as it gets closer and closer to the ground

6 ... you start to feel even more relaxed

5 ... continuing to look at the ant's movement

4 ... feeling the relaxation in every part of your body

3 ... the ant is about to reach the tree roots

2 ...you are getting even more relaxed

1 ... the ant has reached the ground

0 ...You are now comfortably relaxed

Pause

You are now deeply and beautifully relaxed...
And as you focus on the sound of my voice...your imagination opens up even more...

And you notice a long corridor in front of you, with a door at the end of it.

Pause

Just imagine that you are in a long corridor or hallway...and as you notice that...you also notice its walls and the floor...and as you continue to notice that...you allow yourself to relax even more and you move forward towards the door...

Pause

And the door leads you...to a point on the road, where you make a decision about your life. The life that is full of confidence, high self-worth, hope, and positivity or the life that makes you insecure, frustrated, underconfident, and sad. You have a choice to make...an important decision to make. You are at the fork...at a decision point...

One road shows you the life where you see yourself as slim, attractive and confident...whereas the other road shows you the life where you continue to live the life you are already living...perhaps a life with no or less exercise and unhealthy eating.

The road that shows you as slim, confident, and attractive person, living a successful and happy life...is on the right whereas the left road... seems bumpy, dingy, and definitely not happy. Perhaps it's a road of misery...where you see yourself as just the way you are...continuing to live the life you are already living...

And, I wonder if you can take the road to the left and notice what all you see and how you feel.

Pause

Look at your body...your eating habits... your lifestyle...your relationships, do you feel happy seeing yourself on road left?

Pause

And, I wonder if you could see yourself on the same road five years from now... do you see yourself as pleased with yourself? Do you feel healthier or worse?

Get the knowing of it...

Pause

The time has come for you to come back to the fork and the point where you now need to go on the right path of happiness, health, and confidence...and then make a decision…the wise decision…the right decision. And, I know you can do it, because everybody can…

I wonder if you can take that road and see how your life looks like six months from now…the right road shows the active lifestyle…the healthy eating habits… the life where you have taken charge of your life… and emotions… and someone who is determined and focused to achieve daily goals… to achieve the big goal of slimming down and losing weight…isn't it?

Pause

And, I wonder if you could now look at yourself five years from now…living an active lifestyle and I wonder if you could get the knowing of the feelings around that lifestyle…

Do you feel smart about living this kind of life?

Pause

And, now that you have seen both the lives, I wonder if you are ready to make the decision to choose the life that gives you maximum happiness, positivity, hope, confidence, and self-worth…

Pause

And as I count from 3 to 1, you will choose the path that is right for you. The right path that will turn you into a successful, happy, and confident person.

Starting now…

3, 2, and 1.

That's right.
Longer Pause

Confidence and Self Esteem Script

Continuing to go deeper and deeper with every word I say and with every breath you take...you are now getting mentally, physically, and emotionally relaxed and are more receptive to what I say...

Pause

You are now ready to make important changes to your life and to your body that will make you live a happier and fulfilling life.

Pause

And as you continue to listen to me, you become aware of the times you felt low on confidence, perhaps a time in childhood, teens, or from anytime of your life.

You will be able to bring up those memories in black and white....as if you they are like old photo negatives we used to have decades ago.

Pause

And with the power of your mind...you can easily bring up those memories as photo negatives... where someone made you feel low about yourself or perhaps the times where you felt underconfident. Get the knowing of that...

Longer Pause

Notice all those events in the form of old photo negatives coming out of your body... perhaps from different parts of your body ...and moving towards the top of your head.

And as that happens, you feel your body getting lighter and lighter...

You know that they do not belong to you anymore and the today is the day to discard these from your system, your body, your thoughts, your emotions...that's right.

Pause

I don't know if you know that lack of confidence and low self-esteem generally originate from the childhood...perhaps coming from the situations involving teachers...critical parents, peers, friends that make you feel in a certain negative way about yourself.

This happens with most of us but the wise part of us know exactly what to do to be able to let go of these memories to live a better future...and not stay stuck in the past...

And...that part of you is now working for your highest good...

And as I talk to you...the subconscious is now going to make you imagine a bunch of helium balloons coming down from the sky...

Imagine a bunch of helium balloons is coming down to take away those images back to the sky, millions and millions of miles away....

I am going to count from 3 down to 1..and with each count down...the bunch is going to get bigger and bigger as it is going to come closer and closer...to take away that holds no value in your present...

3....2....1

Pause

And I wonder if you could now give away all those black and white photo negatives to the balloons and see them inside the balloons....

Notice how they look inside each balloon...

And, you can barely make out the memories as they look all blurred inside the balloons.

Pause

The time has come to let go of them...and feel liberated...absolutely free...and light...and when the balloons start to take a flight...you will feel free...as if the weight has been lifted...the old baggage...the unwanted...the not needed...that's right...it's all going to go now....away...far away... that's right.

In a moment, you will notice that the bunch of balloons takes a flight back to the universe...back to where it came from.... taking away all that does not solve any purpose.

You are now free from the feelings of low confidence and low self-esteem….as these are the things of past. You had experienced these emotions long time ago and you no longer give them importance as they hold no more importance.

You are free and feeling light mentally, emotionally, and physically.

That's right.

And, I wonder if you could now imagine a color of confidence. The color that resonates with confidence…imagine any color and the moment you imagine that color, you feel confident….

Pause

I wonder if you could now Imagine that color moving into your body and encompassing you from all sides.

As if you are inside the cocoon of confidence, exuding confidence from every part of your body.

And, this confidence helps you to be positive…energetic…happy… and joyful.

With confidence you can achieve all your health goals. That's right…especially the weight you want to be at, it's so much easier now to achieve it. Because you are confident. Absolutely confident about what you want to achieve and who you want to be soon.

You are now confident and this confidence is going to make losing weight easier and simpler. As you start to realise the fact that eating right…and exercising is the way to lose weight. It is 70 percent diet and 30 percent exercise…and if you follow this, you shall start to see the results in no time…

You lose weight when you eat right and exercise to burn off extra calories. This confidence helps you gain control on your eating habits and how you live your life…

If you know what to do, it gets easier to know how to do it… And, I know that you want to lose weight and you will figure out ways how to do that. Isn't it?

With high level of confidence, it gets easier for you to know the ways to achieve your goal weight. And, with every passing day, your self-esteem and self-worth is increasing….

And with every pound you lose, the confidence doubles up and you start to stay even more focused on your goals and this brings the feelings of self-respect…and self-worth. You feel energetic and has the profound sense of well-being.

You are well aware of your self-confidence inside of you…you are self reliant, independent, and absolutely confident. You are full of determination, independence…and you think confidently when making decisions. You are secure and you are ready to transform yourself…fully from inside and outside.

You think and talk confidently…and its visible in your body language…you exude self confidence in your walk and how you behave with people…your friends and family are amazed to see you talk so confidently…

Pause

With this…you are creating a positive reality for yourself…having immense confidence…self worth…self esteem…positivity…and happiness…the inner joy that comes from assertiveness and the ability to make wise decisions…for yourself..

Pause

Because of your positive attitude, positive thinking…and positive way of living…you experience a whole new reality in every area of your life…whether its your work, relationships…or health…

With every passing day…you are getting stronger and stronger in your mind…more assertive…happier…even more confident…that's right…

Pause

You allow yourself to release all the fears and other negative emotions…that serve no purpose…and allow yourself to feel the positive emotions like security, freedom, positivity, happiness, confidence, calmness…contentment…

You are aligned and centred at all times… always looking at living your present day and living it mindfully to achieve the daily goals…living each day beautifully and productively.

You maintain calm and relaxed…focused and mindful. You are confident and secure about everything.

Pause

You are now receptive to all the suggestions for your highest good...to help you achieve your goal weight...

I would like you to now repeat the following affirmations after me in your mind.

I am confident and strong... (5 to 6 second pause)

I have high self esteem... (")

I am secure with myself... (")

I believe in myself ...(")

I am happy and joyous... (")

I take charge of my life...(")

I love myself...(")

I am happiness... (")

I am worthy of love...(")

I attract good things in life...(")

I have unique abilities...(")

I deserve success...(")

I deserve to be fit and healthy...(")

I respect myself...(")

I appreciate myself...(")

People appreciate me...(")

I am wonderful in everyway...(")

I am getting better with every passing day...(")

I deserve to be happy... (")

I am active, energetic, and positive...(")

Boost Your Metabolism

Your body is an expression of who you are inside...who you see yourself as. It shows your discipline and dedication in taking care of yourself. It also influences your sex appeal to others.

Before we start to work on your body, metabolism, exercising, and self-love, I wonder if you know that your outside is the reflection of your inside...to be able to slim down and burn fat, the work needs to be done inside for it to be reflected on the outside.

It is a mix of self-love...eating right...exercise...and proper sleep. And, before you even start taking actions to achieve what you want to achieve...you need to think first. So, I wonder if you can think about all the benefits you will have when achieve your ideal goal weight...

Longer Pause

And all change happens first in the mind... and listening to me only means you are broadening and widening your mind to receive positive information and let that information get absorbed so much so that it is reflected in your actions... Isn't it?

Because what you think, becomes your reality...

And if you think your body to be burning fat with high metabolism, then you will certainly make it your reality...as you see your body into the perfect body sooner than you realise...

To be able to do that I wonder if you can image your perfect body now...that's right... Imagine yourself brimming with vitality and health, just how you want your body and health to be.

Pause

And stay focused on this goal and bring all your focus and attention to this image of yours.... and as you do that, feel the healthy energy starting to get into you and this makes you even calmer and relaxed...

Pause

And imagine yourself at your goal weight... wearing the clothes that are looking great on you...picture yourself looking great.

Pause

Look at your face, your arms, chest, stomach, and legs. Observe every part of your body and once again imagine all the benefits of being at this goal weight.

Longer Pause (10 seconds pause)

You now have a goal in front of you... and you can only accomplish goals... if you have them. And, when you have a goal...you only need to take actions to reach the goals. Isn't it?

And achieving goals is easy and effortless...because you know the benefits of achieving goals and how you can feel, once you have achieved them.

And I wonder if you could feel what you will feel if you achieve the goal of attaining the ideal goal weight. How would you feel?

PAUSE

Stay with the feeling...

And, as you continue to listen to each word I say, you are feeling motivated to be successful at whatever you do.

Eating smaller portions

Exercise and proper diet increase the metabolism... and to be able to do that, you exercise at least 30 minutes every day and eat smaller portions 5- 6 times a day. When you eat frequent smaller portions...you are able to digest better, which in turns boosts the metabolism.

It also helps in stabilizing blood sugar levels and offer nutrients to the body the entire day...

To keep your metabolic rate high...feel less hungry...and have high levels energy, smaller portions of food is the key.

Increase metabolism by eating several smaller meals per day. The idea is to never let yourself get hungry...

And to achieve high metabolism...eat six smaller meals throughout the day instead of having three big meals. Divide your one big meal into two and have it in the gap of two to three hours. It is easy and this way you will never starve yourself...and save yourself from binge eating.

Pause

The way you will accomplish this is to eat healthy nutritious meals and eat healthy nutritious snacks in between those meals keeping yourself satisfied throughout the day. Include fruits and more salads in the diet to eat healthy and keep the stomach full with smaller portions.

And with this, you can notice that all body parts and organs are functioning at the optimal level... with a thought to improve the body through nutritious diet and exercising.

With every passing day...you can notice increase in your energy levels and the metabolism is becoming aligned with your needs.

You consciously and subconsciously reduce the portion size...to be able to eat the right amount of nutritious food...and you eat foods that are good for your health.

And this makes you feel so much relaxed and calm... as you continue to listen to each word I say.

Your metabolism gets adjusted when your body is at rest...you feel a sense of peace and calm within you and because of all the improvements taking place in your mind, your are able to pump more oxygen in your lungs and your heartbeat becomes steadier and breathing becomes natural.

This only means that your nervous system is beginning to function more appropriately...and all the organs are working harmoniously inside your body. That's right.

You are a confident person and believe in yourself...You can effortlessly and easily release all the extra weight to reach your ideal goal weight.

Pause

You are a lovable and confident person...you will eat only when you are hungry and not eat foods to pass time or eat when there is some emotional trigger... You will no longer food to give you the comforting feeling... because that only means you give all the power to the food and then the extra or junk food makes you be what you do not want to be.

So... you take charge of your life and take charge of your body.

And the more you do it... the better control you have on your eating and exercise habits. You notice that with every passing day... you are becoming focused on your goal and you take actions accordingly to accomplish it.

Pause

And now I wonder if you could imagine yourself as an attractive woman and as you begin to act and walk like a healthy and attractive woman, you manifest it...and make it your reality.

With paying attention to the portions and thoughts before taking extra food...you allow yourself to eat less and feel confident.

Pause

Imagine just deciding on eating smaller portions can already make you feel good about yourself...isn't it?

Through this recording, you are able to bring satisfaction which leads to relaxation and brings you a healthy, attractive, and slimmer body….

Get Rid of the Sweet Tooth

And you focus on the sound of my voice and allow yourself to go even deeper with every breath you take…and with every word I say.

And all these words sink into your subconscious mind effortlessly and you begin to feel even more comfy and relaxed….

If your food habits also include having desserts, sweetened drinks, and other sugary stuff then you may have difficulty in losing weight faster.

Pause

And you are listening to me because you want to get rid of the sweet tooth you have and end the sugar cravings forever. Isn't it?

Pause

And, I wonder if you can look into your mouth with your mind's eye for that tooth that makes you crave sweets and you know because of that you may not lose weight easily.

Longer Pause

And you have found it….and the time has come to talk to the tooth and understand the purpose of it…

Perhaps the purpose of the tooth is to eat sugars…and you know there are natural sugars in fruits that can satiate the tooth…without affecting your body.

Because you love yourself and are excited to meet your weight loss goals and be at your ideal goal weight…you are going to make a contract with the sweet tooth that it will only be happy with the sugars coming from fresh fruits and vegetables. You can substitute white sugar with raw honey or jaggery…that will make the tooth and you happy.

This will be a win - win situation for you both…and I know you can convince the sweet tooth…can't you?

Pause

You know that sugary fruits and artificially sweetened drinks and foods will convert the sugar into fat...that will harden the arteries, adding fat to the body, and also rotting the teeth.

Sweet Tooth is a part of your body and it is a small part of you...you cannot make it so big in your system...that it controls your eating habits and make you gain weight...isn't it?

You will turn the sweet tooth into a healthy tooth that is happy having natural sugars and you will be aware of all the foods having natural sugars, so that you only have those...and satiate the desire of the healthy tooth.

And the healthy tooth only craves healthy foods, natural sugars, lots of water, fruits and vegetables, and whole grains.

Pause

I wonder if you could go back to the time when you first loved having sugary foods...perhaps a time when you were much younger...

Longer Pause

And the adult part of you that is listening to this audio, has the capability to go to that time when the younger self of yours started loving sweets, perhaps chocolates, candies, and similar foods. Maybe your parents gave them to you to pacify you...

The time has come to meet the younger self and talk to the child about the long term bad effects of having too much sweet and sugary stuff...

And also tell the child about the benefits of having natural sugars...the effects it has on skin, gut, and overall mood.

I would like you to speak to the child as if it were your own...and talk to the child...

Longer Pause

And, once you have spoken to the child...take the child from that time back to this time....as I count from 3 to 1.

3, 2, and 1...

And, you are now back with the child...and the child knows all the benefits of having natural sugars and all the disadvantages of having artificial sweetened foods or foods loaded with sugar.

In a moment, you both will become one with each other as one individual who does not crave sugar anymore...and only loves to have natural sugars...

Imagine yourself now integrating into each other...make the child reside in your heart...and see yourself as one person who is excited to stick to the weight loss plan to reach the weight loss goal.

Longer Pause

You know sweet drinks and sweetened foods with sugar are like poison to your body.

And with this awareness, you are able to spot sugary foods easily and stop yourself from eating and drinking them...instead you think wisely and choose foods with natural sugars to satiate the craving and make yourself and the healthy tooth happy and satiated.

Pause

You are now one...someone who looks for sugar only in fruits...and you enjoy having fruits and vegetables.

And, now imagine yourself at the ideal goal weight...looking absolutely stunning...and attractive.

You know you have reached this goal only by making changes to your diet and including a regular exercise regimen in your routine....

How does it feel to be this successful?

Pause

LOW CARB DIET

And, I wonder… if you could now join me in a fun exercise where you will imagine a platter full of delicious and colourful fruits and vegetables.

Pause

As you take a look at the platter… you start to salivate as they look so fresh. They are farm fresh, tender…delicious and vibrant. Take a closer look at the fruits and vegetables…look at the skin of fruits and veggies, touch and smell them. Perhaps there is a bright green broccoli that is rich in protein and the vibrant carrot, full of vitamins…

Pause

You pick up what you really like and get attracted to, and bite into the deliciousness and freshness. And, as you do that… you feel the taste buds dancing with joy…

Longer Pause

You overlooked all these foods and their goodness from coming into your body before and today is the day to realise the value of these foods… You just made a decision to switch to a low-carb diet…another great and wise decision to live a healthy and active life.

Pause

You eat healthy foods to not only be healthy and to lose weight but also to be mentally alert. Healthy foods make you get through the day effortlessly and with lean proteins, fruits, veggies, and whole grains…you get minerals, vitamins and nutrients to keep yourself in optimal health….

Because it is important to balance carbohydrates and proteins, you take whole grains and lean proteins that are excellent source of energy…Vegetables, fruits, and whole grains have fibre in them that keeps you full for longer… The darker the veggies the more nutrients they have….

And you think of having a beautiful and glowy skin with the kind of body you desire…it is going to be a complete transformation…and you are so looking forward to living a life full of confidence, high self-esteem, active and slim body, and clear skin...and all this is possible with the wise decisions you have already made today...

Longer Pause

By making your first steps into the world of healthy foods...you experienced the joy of eating mindfully...of taking care of your diet as well as your body...thus promoting a healthy mind and body. You feel fitter, lighter, slimmer and overall great. That's right.

And I wonder, if you could now imagine that these low carb foods are entering your stomach. And because they are low on carbohydrates....low levels of insulin are secreted and because of the low calorie or low carb diet...the body uses stored up fat for energy and leaves no room for fat backlog...which helps you to lose weight.

Pause

And with your great imagination, I wonder if you could, Imagine how clean your stomach looks from inside, take a closer look at the intestines, it's a happy stomach...isn't it?

And, with light and happy stomach, you feel so energised and full of vibrancy...

Pause

You now know the advantages of eating low calorie diet and some of the benefits are weight loss...fat reduction...high levels of energy...and livelier you.

And, I wonder if you can now tick off the low calorie and non- starchy, protein rich foods like lean meat, fish, beans, succulent fruits and vegetables...in your mind somewhere...

Pause

And that only means that ...from today on, you will be eating more of these foods to keep your stomach and yourself happy. Absolutely loving each smaller meal and moving towards your ideal goal weight.

Pause

You eat mindfully, embracing protein rich…low carb foods. Your diet includes colourful fruits, vegetables. You consciously make efforts to reduce the portion size and increase the frequency of meals to six meals per day.

You drink at least eight glasses of water every day. Eating right is your new everyday goal to reach the bigger goal of release extra fat and weight to be able to reach your goal weight.

Pause

And I would like you to repeat the suggestions in your mind after me…

I eat healthy foods (4 seconds pauses)

I eat smaller portions (4 seconds pauses)

I exercise regularly (4 seconds pauses)

I am conscious of my eating habits (4 seconds pauses)

I eat mindfully (4 seconds pauses)

I exercise regularly (4 seconds pauses)

Pause

Be Motivated to Exercise

And you are now wondering how much exercise you are getting everyday and you know to be able to fasten the metabolism and lose weight easily, you need to also exercise in addition to eating right...

And I wonder if you could imagine a control room somewhere in your brain...perhaps it looks like a room with wires, knobs, buttons with lights flickering...

Longer Pause

You look at the control panel and you know to be able to control the functions in your mind and body, you need to fix something in here...

I don't know what that is ....but you know...

That's right..

Pause

You continue to look around in the control room and find a knob for exercise...and it has numbers around the knob from 0 to 10...perhaps the knob's indicator is set at a lower number and that causes you to procrastinate when it comes to exercising.

To be able to stay motivated and exercise every day...you may want to turn up the knob to a higher number...

Pause

And this only means that you will be excited every day to finish your workout session...because with every workout session you feel happier and confident about yourself...

This is one way to boost confidence and feel amazing...

And, perhaps there is a light flickering in the control room and that is the light of procrastination...and its flickering only means that its activated...and to be able to switch it off...you may want to cut the power cord....

You have the equipment to cut it now...

Cut now...that's right..

Pause

You have cut all cords with procrastination...because it never helped you...but only made you feel sad and guilty of not taking actions..

And, now you are free...liberated from the ties of procrastination...

Pause

You now start to wonder which exercise program will help you and you may begin to think that exercise is all about having a regimen that includes cardiovascular activity, some weight lifting, and stretching.

Pause

You begin to wonder that how many steps do you walk everyday...perhaps you need to walk a bit more and have a pedometer on your phone or some app to track the steps...

Pause

And you begin to feel active and energetic as soon as you finish walking 5000 steps a day. You add some more exercises to the routine...perhaps few Yoga Asanaas, pilates...or aerobics....and your mind choose the exercises that will bring maximum benefit to your body and help you achieve your weight goal really fast.

And with every passing day, you begin to realise that it's so much easier to exercise just like how you brush your teeth or take a shower and make exercise a part of your routine....effortless..

Pause

Sometimes you just stretch your legs and arms to feel relaxed and perhaps do some Pilates or aerobics by following an instructor on a video.

You can even just dance freestyle every day on your favorite dance numbers because the idea is to move your body and let the heart race to feel the burn and sweat to lose weight much faster...

And, I would like you to say the following suggestions in your mind after me..

I exercise everyday

(Pause for 5 seconds)

I move your body more

(Pause for 5 seconds)

I set exercise goals for every day

(Pause for 5 seconds)

I enjoy your exercise program

(Pause for 5 seconds)

I sweat and feel great

(Pause for 5 seconds)

I look forward to my exercise session every morning

Say No to Emotional Eating

And, as you continue to focus on the sound of my voice...I wonder if you could imagine a big projector screen in front of you....

Pause

And on the screen...you see yourself just before the time the emotional eating started. Perhaps it was few months ago or....a few years ago. I know you can easily access that memory, because everybody can.

Pause

Because a part of you can go through all the relevant memories that led you to start eating emotionally or when emotions overpowered you so much so, that you looked forward to eating food to feel happy and comfortable.

Pause

And, as that part of you looks for these memories... it can find the hidden emotion and you know many people with emotional eating issues discover that events led to emotional or comfort eating cause us to feel shame or guilt...and while looking for the events and emotions, you can easily begin...to notice how the series of events move backwards on the screen and then move forward like a fast forward.

Pause

That's right... you notice this happening quite a few times, until the events related to emotional eating get blurred and the images get totally distorted.

Longer Pause

And let the emotions related to those events simply get distorted with the images and you begin to form new coping strategies for success and achievement.

Pause

And as you continue to go deeper and deeper... listening to each word I say, I wonder if you know that the subconscious mind learns much faster than you can imagine....

Pause

And, that is why, you are now receptive to every positive word I say that will help you achieve a slimmer and fitter body...

I wonder if you could know the purpose of a refrigerator and the purpose is to keep the vegetables, fruits, milk, eggs, and much more fresh. And, similarly, the purpose of a vehicle is to take us to different places...isn't it?

Similarly, can you know the purpose of your feelings?

Pause

And, maybe you are struggling to know the purpose...

Sometimes, feelings of boredom's purpose is to make us overeat and the feelings of sadness's purpose is to again make us order in and eat junk food...

Sometimes, feelings of anxiety can cause us to overeat...and what action we take is a reaction to a feeling.

And overeating or eating junk food only makes us feel happy for a temporary moment and then causes us to feel guilty...and that's the beginning of a vicious cycle...

The feelings of guilt may again lead us to eat more... and then ultimately make us overweight...

Pause

So, eating in response to a feeling does not satisfy hunger...it only give a temporary relief and distracts us from a particular negative feeling.

And, as you continue to listen to what I say...you now know that you did not have any idea what needs to be done with the feelings. And, some people ignore them, some hide them, and some people distract themselves... by eating more.

And I wonder if you know that how the alarms goes off when you have to go for a meeting...indicating you to get up on time to reach office. If you do not pay attention to it, you may miss going to the meeting, which may have other consequences.

So similarly....alarm as an indicator asks you to take an action, but the action need to be the right action, which is to get up and start getting ready for the meeting....

And not take the action gets you in the loop of feeling the negative feelings again like frustration or guilt.

So, anytime a negative feeling arises, you need to think twice before taking an action. If you are feeling lonely, instead of picking up the phone to order food in, you may want to pick the phone to call your family or friends...

Pause

If you are feeling sad or stressed, instead of overeating... you may want to practice coping strategies like watching something funny... taking deep breaths, journaling the thoughts, or distracting your mind to do something else and feel a different feeling...

From now on, whenever you get a feeling and it's not hunger, you show yourself a red light- the stop light where you think twice and take the right action to not get into the loop of negative feelings. I know you can do it, because everybody can.

You are more aware of when you are actually physically hungry as compared to when you are hungry to satisfy emotions.

Pause

It gets easier for you to recognise feelings just before eating that is it the stomach that is hungry or the mind?

If it's the mind, then how can I distract my mind and take different actions to be able to divert myself from eating.

You may want to go for a walk or have a tall glass of water

Or talk to your family or play with your pet...

There are many ways to divert your mind to be able to take right actions and not eat in response of emotions.

Pause

And, when you are in control of your emotions, you get pleasure and satisfaction and you feel even more confident about yourself.

You are more ready than ever to feel happy, positive, fit, and confident...

And, with this feeling, you begin to realise that you can be calm, relaxed, and think wisely when it comes to taking actions.

Even when the challenges come, you are calm and relaxed and take actions when you have given much thought to it...

Your confidence continues to increase with every passing day, knowing you deserve to feel healthy and fit at your ideal goal weight.

Pause

You then use every other action that stops you from overeating or eating unhealthy foods.

And I want you to repeat the following suggestions in your mind after me...

I am conscious of my feelings

Pause

I am mindful of my actions

Pause

I love myself and think twice before taking actions

Pause

I am confident and believe in myself...

Heal Your Body

I wonder... if you could now imagine a beautiful and warm golden energy coming from the Sun. The beautiful Sun that gives the planet all the light and energy...

And imagine the energy or Sun light touching your head like a sharp beam ...

The energy from the Sun is positive and healing and you can feel it moving into the top of your head...feel it inside of your head and perhaps with your third eye...see it moving into every cell and fibre of it.

That's right.

Imagine all the thoughts about past that no longer serve purpose and only make you feel negative in a certain way are moving out of your head... All those limiting beliefs about yourself... that you created or perhaps the labels given to you by others. All of those have no value in your life...and all those can't stop you from moving ahead in life.

Pause

As soon as the golden healing light touches every part of your mind, the beliefs about your body that you created at some point in life...the negative beliefs... those will simply go away.

Because the positive energy from the Sun clears your mind of all the negative thoughts and limiting beliefs that have no more value and serve no purpose...you allow yourself to let that happen...because this is the time to love yourself even more.

Pause

And it starts to further move down...towards your eyes...making you feel even more relaxed as you continue to listen to each word I say.

Further down to your facial muscles...cheeks, upper lips...jaws, and chin. Relaxing every part and muscle in your face...feeling the sense of calm in every part of your face.

And this happens, you begin to feel very comfortable in your own skin and start to love yourself more and more...

You now imagine the beautiful Sun's energy moving into your shoulders…taking away unwanted burdens that you may have.

Feel the energy into your shoulders, giving them all the comfort as you notice the energy moving into them with your mind's eye. Feel all the stress and burden taken away as the energy reaches your shoulders…

Pause

And, allow that beautiful golden energy, the comforting energy to touch your heart chakra, the center of your chest, and that's the seat of self-love. Imagine it moving down from your shoulders to the center of your chest…

Pause

And, I wonder if you could imagine activating the heart chakra and visualize the golden color turning green and moving in a clock-wise direction…Imagine this chakra moving like a fan or wheel in a clockwise direction…and this only means that you have started to love yourself even more. That's right.

Pause

And as you notice it moving like a fan or wheel … you notice all the blockages in the heart chakra to be simply melting away. These blockages are stuck emotions related to past events or perhaps they are some worries. And, clearing the chakra and activating it with the green energy only means you are now activating the heart chakra to be able to bring self-love.

Longer Pause

The energy now moves into your arms, relaxing your arm muscles. Reaching every cell and fiber of your arms…making your arms and hands so very relaxed…that's right.

Pause

It now further moves down to your waist…and torso…and as this happens, you feel the sense of deep appreciation for yourself.

Pause

And as it continues to move down into your hips and thighs, you drift deeper and deeper into self-love. That's right.

And you can notice the golden light making its way into the wrists and fingers…

And as that happens, you tighten your fists and say to yourself. – "I can do it" That's right.

You can do it.

You can achieve all the goals that you have set for yourself on this weight loss journey...

Pause

The everyday goals to eat healthy to achieve the big goal of achieving your ideal weight. Isn't it?

You can see the energy moving into your feet and toes. Making you feel so relaxed, calm and at the same time positive and energetic...just like sun.

And you feel so determined to achieve the weight loss goals. I know you can do it because everybody can.

Pause

You now notice your whole body filled with golden healing energy...

This also has the power to melt the fat stored in your every part of your body...that perhaps make you look overweight or chubby...

Imagine all the fat getting melted...

you have the power to get rid of all the accumulated fat...

Longer Pause

And in a moment, you will notice that the light of self-love is melting the fat stored in your body. And with every breath you take and with every rise and fall of your chest, you can easily visualize fat melting away from your thighs, hips, stomach and other body part that has extra fat.

Longer Pause

You can do it

Pause

You know exactly how to lose weight

Pause

You are smart and very intelligent to make right decisions

Pause

You take actions every day to achieve daily goals

Pause

You love yourself even more with every passing day

Pause

You love your body

Pause

You are mindful and enjoy the present moment

Pause

You are slimming now

You are slimming Now

And, as you continue to relax even more… with every breath you take and with every word I say…it is even more easier for you feel and see what we are going to do…

My words are getting embedded in your mind… for your highest good…for you to achieve your weight loss goal. You have decided to not only lose weight but also tone and slim the body to look your best…

Pause

Because of the extra weight and fat, you may have experienced situations where you felt uncomfortable about your body, whether it was wearing a short dress or going into the pool. Because of the extra weight, you could not wear your favorite dresses and could not feel comfy in the clothes you were wearing. Isn't it?

Pause

And…you may have felt embarrassment, anger, frustration, shame, insecurity and sadness because of the extra weight you had been carrying.

Imagine if this continues to go on, how would you feel after a year or two years? Maybe sad again. Isn't it?

Longer Pause

You do not have to worry about living the same life after a year or two years because you are listening to me and you have already decided to change your body and change your life. Isn't it?

But now, there is no chance of going back to that life… living those negative emotions every day. You now know how important it is to lose weight and get slim.

Pause

You are ready to change… because slimming will transform every area of your life… Your health…your relationships…your work…and of course the most important area of self. You will have a beautiful relationship with yourself.

With new attitude, you have new hopes and positivity to take your life to the next level.

The moment you start to slim down and lose weight…you feel hopeful and positive and life seems so much better.

You are hopeful and it does not matter…how much you tried in the past, you know that this time, you are going to achieve your ideal goal weight. Every new action towards your goal will free you from your past and in no time, you will see the results in your body.

Pause

You are ready to make small changes in the area of your health… Some of the small changes are eating right… having a control on emotions…and exercising regularly.

And I wonder if you can now paint yourself on a canvas, which is hung on an easel. The painting is of your new slim body, the perfect silhouette, beautiful and attractive.

Paint yourself with a healthier body having a positive vibe and energy.

I am going to stay quiet for a few moments, so that you can paint yourself with the clothes that you would want to wear, looking absolutely gorgeous and confident.

Longer Pause

And, with your imagination…you have the capability to enter into the canvas and enter the woman you have just drawn and painted.

Imagine yourself on the canvas, looking absolutely gorgeous, confident, hopeful, positive, having a slim and attractive body.

You may want to feel your legs, arms, torso, and chest. See how it feels to be slim. Amazing, isn't it?

With this, you are absolutely sure that to feel amazing, you need to have a slim body. You know that you must change now.

These changes that you are making will have positive effects on your body and life. Imagine what it would be like doing other important things in your life in your new beautiful body.

Feel the confidence you will have once you have achieved the desired body shape and weight. Imagine doing the things you desire to do like adventure sports and other similar such activities that you have always wanted to do but stopped yourself from doing because of the extra weight your carried.

And this how you will live the rest of your life, absolutely confident, positive, with high self-esteem.

I am going to count from 1 to 5 and with each count up, the feelings of confidence, hope, positivity, and self-esteem will double up.

1, 2, 3, 4, and 5.

That's right.

And, say to yourself – " I am slimming" and notice how amazing you feel when you say these words – " I am slimming"

And, every time in future, you want to remind yourself of the journey you are on. Simply say – I am slimming and you will be able to bring back the feelings of confidence, high self-esteem, positivity and hope.

Pause

Anytime, you feel like overeating or skipping the exercise program, say the words I am slimming, and you will be back to the thoughts of losing weight and take the right actions.

Reinforcement Script

And, you continue to drift down...deeper and deeper into...a beautiful comfy feeling...focusing on the sound of my voice and focusing on the goal of achieving your ideal weight.

It is so wonderful to feel relaxed and drift down... into a lovely feeling and as you do so, you can really start to feel good and enjoy this calming space. So perfect to be here and listen to me.

And...you can drop all your tensions and your body knows how to feel relaxed and good and with every breath you take, you find it easier and easier to fall further into this deep relaxation. And your body exactly knows how to feel happy and good and feel relaxed.

Pause

So, just let go and go with the flow and think about nothing, nothing at all as all you need to do is to simply relax and let go...

Pause

And congratulations on your decision to live your life in a healthier way...you have made the decision and commitment to yourself and with the help of hypnosis, we can use the positive reinforcement to help you maintain the motivation to eat healthy and exercise regularly to achieve your ideal goal weight and body.

And because of old habits...you know that you are creating issues for your health and body. And with healthy habits and exercise... you can turn it around and be someone that you always wanted to be. Fit, slimmer, and healthy.

Pause

You overcame all your old limiting beliefs and behaviours and you took charge of your life and this makes you feel great about yourself. Isn't it?

And from today, you look forward a successful future where you see yourself as a positive, healthy, joyful, and confident person. You see yourself as successful.

With every passing day...your old way of living fades away as you continue to move forward through the tunnel and leave behind all that does not serve any purpose and does not belong to you and in front you notice light...the new life awaits. The brighter life, the healthier life is waiting for you.

You are excited and curious to look forward to a successful and healthy life.

And you can achieve the life you desire right now only when you are motivated and determined.

With every passing day, the motivation and determination are getting stronger and stronger.

Pause

You are determined to put healthy nutritious food in your mouth and you chew it at least 10 times. You drink at least 8 glasses of water. You exercise at least 30 minutes every day.

And because you need to take care of your mind, you also need to take care of you mind, to look beautiful inside out. And, that is why you also start to look after your mind. You think happy and remain in the present moment.

Pause

You practice mindfulness and focus on what is at hand instead of thinking about what has gone or what is coming.

Mindfulness or focusing on the here …and now allows you to be positive and keeps you focused on your weight loss journey. You think positive and feel positive which leads to positive actions.

Pause

You are so happy to have made a decision and commitment to a healthier life. A healthier you await you and in no time, you will be able to meet her soon. The slimmer and happier you. Isn't it?

You are proud of yourself and you deserve to experience the feelings of accomplishment… and with every passing day, you are getting even more determined to meet the everyday goals of eating healthy and exercising regularly.

And as you continue to take actions and see the results, you also inspire people around you. From family and friends, to colleagues and relatives, everyone is surprised to see your determination and they ask you the secrets of losing weight.

Pause

You feel so good already that you are able to accomplish the long-desired goal to lose weight and you can feel the difference in your body and you feel in your old clothes. They are getting lose on you.

Pause

You are excited to change the wardrobe once you reach the ideal goal weight and look your best, aligned to the latest fashion.

Now imagine yourself again at the goal weight you want to be at and see the clothes you are wearing.

Pause

Feel how you are feeling, perhaps liberated, confident, excited, healthier, and happier. Isn't it?

Suggestions/Affirmations

1. You are becoming slimmer and stronger (5 seconds Pause)
2. You are mindful of eating (Same as above)
3. You exercise regularly (Same as above)
4. You sleep well every night and take at least 6 hours of deep sleep (Same as above)
5. You enjoy eating green, dark leafy vegetables (Same as above)
6. Your body is becoming slimmer with every passing day (Same as above)
7. You are in control of your life (Same as above)
8. You have taken charge of your life and body (Same as above)
9. You feel good when you eat healthy and exercise regularly (Same as above)
10. Your body gets rid of extra fat (Same as above)
11. Your love yourself with every passing day (Same as above)
12. You are motivated to achieve your ideal goal weight (Same as above)
13. You avoid high calorie food (Same as above)
14. You enjoy smaller portions of food (Same as above)
15. You chew eat mouthful atleast 10 times and relish the flavors (Same as above)
16. You eat fresh fruits and savor the flavors (Same as above)
17. You look forward to your exercise session every day (Same as above)
18. You are positive (Same as above)
19. You are focused on your daily actions and daily goals (Same as above)
20. You see yourself having the ideal body and weight (Same as above)
21. You stay focused on this weight loss journey (Same as above)
22. You enjoy the taste of fresh fruits (Same as above)
23. You enjoy the taste of veggies (Same as above)
24. You include lean proteins and skimmed milk in your diet (Same as above)
25. You enjoy the taste of salads (Same as above)
26. Your body is becoming slimmer (Same as above)
27. Your stomach and hips are becoming smaller (Same as above)
28. You are getting stronger and leaner (Same as above)
29. You gain muscle and lose weight (Same as above)
30. You feel stronger and stronger with every passing day (Same as above)
31. Your trust your body and it gets easier and easier to trust it (Same as above)
32. Your health is improving with every passing day (Same as above)
33. Making small changes are becoming so much easier for you (Same as above)
34. You are patient and believe in yourself (Same as above)
35. You believe that you will achieve the weight loss goal (Same as above)

36. Letting go of past is easier (Same as above)
37. You are in control of your emotions (Same as above)
38. You are focused and determined (Same as above)
39. You are full of energy (Same as above)
40. You are the creator of your own future (Same as above)
41. You believe your strengths and capabilities (Same as above)
42. You are capable to lose weight (Same as above)
43. You love and accept yourself (Same as above)
44. You are full of self-love (Same as above)
45. You give your body all the nutrients it needs (Same as above)
46. Every day of exercise and eating right food makes you even more confident (Same as above)
47. You are confident (Same as above)
48. You have high self-worth (Same as above)
49. Your love for yourself increases with every passing day (Same as above)
50. You are focused on your weight loss journey (Same as above)

All these suggestions are firmly embedded in your sub-conscious mind and with every passing day, getting stronger and stronger with every passing day, hour, minute.

Waking Up

In a moment, I am going to count you up from one to five and with each count up, you will be back in the present moment and wide awake. Feeling fully refreshed and looking forward to the new you.

Starting now at one, two, three, coming slowly back, four – eyelids beginning to flutter and five – eyes open wide awake.

www.ingramcontent.com/pod-product-compliance
Lightning Source LLC
Chambersburg PA
CBHW080628030426
42336CB00018B/3114